Lean ᴄ Cookbook

Very Simple Super Fast, and Tasty Recipes to Lose Weight Easily Without Stress Following this Healthy Guide.

LARA LEWIS

By reading this document, the reader agrees that under no circumstances is the author responsible for any losses, direct or indirect, which are incurred as a result of the use of information contained within this document, including, but not limited to, — errors, omissions, or inaccuracies.

TABLE OF CONTENT

Introduction

What is a Lean & Green meal?

A lean, green meal includes 5 to 7 ounces of cooked lean protein plus three servings of non-starchy vegetables and

up to two servings of healthy fats, depending on lean protein choices. Enjoy your Lean & Green meal at any time of the day - whatever works best for your schedule.

Incorporate up to two servings of healthy fats into your Lean & Green meal each day. Healthy fats are important because they help yours the body absorbs vitamins such as A, D, E, and K. They also help your gallbladder function properly.

The lean and green meal must have the following essential ingredients to keep it healthy and safe:

Seafood:

Fish is the best to have in any weight loss regimen because it is free of saturated fat and brings a lot of nutritional value to the table. You can have all kinds of fish and seafood in this diet including halibut, salmon, trout, lobster, tuna, shrimp, crab, and scallops, etc.

Meat:

The lean and green diet allows only 85 percent lean meat on a diet; whether it's chicken, beef, turkey, lamb, pork, and ground beef, it must all be lean. Lean meat has a lower fat content, making it great for keeping calorie intake in check.

Eggs:

Eggs are high in protein and low in carbohydrates; this is what makes eggs suitable for this diet.

Soy products:

In soy products, tofu is the only product allowed in the diet because it is processed and the calorie content is suitable for the lean diet.

Fats:

Not all fats are healthy and there are a handful of options you need to try in this diet, which includes most olive vegetable oil, walnut oil, canola oil, flaxseed oil.

Low-Carb Vegetables:

Focus on all green vegetables for this diet. With the exception of potatoes, sweet potatoes, yellow squash, and beets, you can try every other vegetable on this diet, including kale, spinach, cucumbers, etc.

RECIPES

Tomato Kale and Egg Muffin

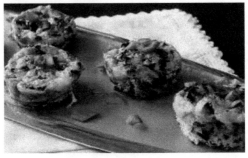

Prep Time: 15 mins **Cook Time:** 20 mins **Total Time:** 35 mins

MAKES 4 SERVINGS

INGREDIENTS

- 3/4 cup low-fat Greek yogurt
- 1 cup egg whites
- 1/3 teaspoon salt
- 1 1/2 cups chopped roma tomatoes
- 1 (10-oz) package chopped kale
- 2 oz feta cheese, crumbled

INSTRUCTIONS

1. Preheat your oven to 375 F.
2. Combine the egg whites, yogurt, cheese, and salt in a bowl.
3. Add in the kale and chopped tomatoes
4. Lightly spray 20-cup muffin tin and pour the mixture into each well.

5. Bake the muffin for about 25 minutes or until s toothpick inserted in the center comes out clean.

Cajun Pork Chops and Spinach Salad

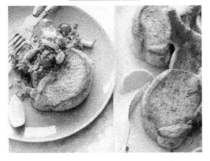

Prep Time: 15 mins **Cook Time:** 20 mins **Total Time:** 35 mins

MAKES 4 SERVINGS

INGREDIENTS

- ➢ 28-ounce pork chops
- ➢ 1 tablespoon Cajun seasoning
- ➢ 1 cup fresh tomatoes, chopped
- ➢ 1 lemon, juiced
- ➢ salt and pepper to tast
- ➢ Lemon wedges for garnish

INSTRUCTIONS

1. Season the pork chops with the Cajun seasoning, 1/8 teaspoon salt, and 1/8 teaspoon pepper.
2. Set aside to marinate for about 25 minutes. (The longer the better)

3. Cook the pork in a preheated oven at 450 F for 10 minutes.
4. Meanwhile, heat the water in a pot. Add in the spinach and cook until wilted.
5. Transfer the spinach to a bowl. Add in the tomatoes, lemon juice, the remaining salt, and pepper.
6. Serve pork chops with spinach salad and lemon wedge(s) by the side.

Skinny Rarebit

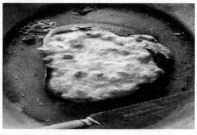

Prep Time: 5 mins **Cook Time:** 6 mins **Total Time:** 11 mins

MAKES 1 SERVINGS

INGREDIENTS

- ➤ 1 x 3 oz. mushrooms, wiped clean
- ➤ 1 teaspoon of mustard
- ➤ 1 level tbsp Philadelphia light
- ➤ salt and pepper to tast

INSTRUCTIONS

1. Grill the mushrooms as above, then spread the tops with the mustard, using the back of a teaspoon. Divide the cheese between the mushrooms in an even layer. Grill for 3 minutes. Season and serve while still hot.

2. As this version is so low in cals, you could serve with a 2 oz. slice of wholemeal toast or a Warburton's Thin.

3. You could use pesto instead of mustard (1/2 teaspoon of bottled pesto is around 23 calories, depending on brand),

and top with a 2 oz. pre-sliced piece of light Cheddar, crumbled.

Tuscan Bean Suop

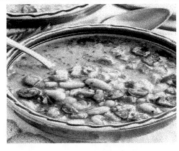

Prep Time: 15 mins **Cook Time:** 20 mins **Total Time:** 35 mins

MAKES 4 SERVINGS

INGREDIENTS

- ➤ 2 slices Parma ham
- ➤ 1 onion
- ➤ 2 carrots,
- ➤ 2 sticks celery,
- ➤ 14 oz. tin mixed beans,
- ➤ 2 large tomatoes
- ➤ 1 litres of chicken stock
- ➤ 2.6 oz. savoy cabbage
- ➤ 0.3 oz. Parmesan cheese, grated

INSTRUCTIONS

1. Preheat the grill. Lightly oil a baking sheet with cooking spray. Place the ham on the baking sheet and grill for about 6 minutes, until crisp. Remove and set aside to coo

2. Spray a large non-stick saucepan with cooking spray, add the onion, carrots and celery and water to help the vegetables steam and fry for 5 minutes.

3. Stir i n the beans, tomatoes and hot stock, bring to the boil, cover with a lid and simmer for 10 minutes. Stir in the cabbage and simmer for 5 minutes, or until just tender.

4. Spoon into serving bowls and scatter with the Parmesan and crumble over the crispy ham.

Crispy Apples

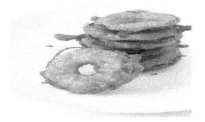

Prep Time: 10 mins **Cook Time:** 10 mins **Total Time:** 20 mins

MAKES 4 SERVINGS

INGREDIENTS

- ➢ 2 tbsp. of cinnamon powder
- ➢ 5 apples
- ➢ ½ tbsp. of nutmeg powder
- ➢ 1 tbsp. of maple syrup
- ➢ ½ cup of water
- ➢ 4 tbsp. of butter
- ➢ ¼ cup of flour
- ➢ ¾ cup of oats
- ➢ ¼ cup of brown sugar

INSTRUCTIONS

1. Get the apples in a pan, put in nutmeg, maple syrup, cinnamon, and water.
2. Mix in butter with flour, sugar, salt, and oat, turn, put a

spoonful of the blend over apples, get into the air fryer and cook at 350°F for 10 minutes.

3. Serve while warm.

Zucchini Noodles with Creamy Avocado Pesto

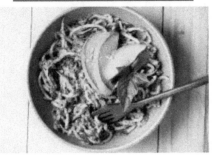

Prep Time: 10 mins **Cook Time:** 20 mins **Total Time:** 30 mins

MAKES 4 SERVINGS

INGREDIENTS

- 1 tbsp. of olive oil
- 6 oz. of avocado
- 1 basil leaves
- 3 garlic cloves
- 1/3 oz. of pine nuts
- 2 tbsp. of lemon juice
- ½ tsp. of salt
- ¼ tsp. of black pepper

INSTRUCTIONS

1. Spiralize the courgettes and set them aside on paper towels to absorb the surplus water.

2. In a food processor, put avocados, juice basil leaves, garlic, pine nuts, and sea salt and pulse until chopped. Then put vegetable oil in a slow stream till emulsified and creamy.
3. Drizzle vegetable oil in a skillet over medium-high heat and put zucchini noodles, cooking for about 2 minutes till tender.
4. Put zucchini noodles in an enormous bowl and toss with avocado pesto. Season with cracked pepper and a little Parmesan and serve.

Ricotta Ramekins

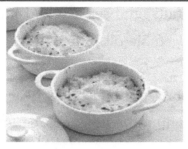

Prep Time: 10 mins **Cook Time:** 1hr **Total Time:** 1 hr 10 mins

MAKES 4 SERVINGS

INGREDIENTS

- ➢ 6 eggs, whisked
- ➢ 1 and ½ pounds of ricotta cheese, soft
- ➢ ½ pound of stevia
- ➢ 1 teaspoon of vanilla extract
- ➢ ½ teaspoon of baking powder
- ➢ Cooking spray

INSTRUCTIONS

1. In a bowl, mix eggs with ricotta and the other ingredients, except for the cooking spray, and whisk well.
2. Grease 4 ramekins with the cooking spray, pour the ricotta cream in each and bake at 360 degrees F for 1 hour.
3. Serve cold.

Chicken Lo Mein

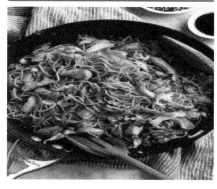

Prep Time: 15 mins **Cook Time:** 30 mins **Total Time:** 35 mins

MAKES 4 SERVINGS

INGREDIENTS

- 2 tbsp. + 2 tsp. of sesame oil, divided
- 790g boneless. skinless chicken breasts, sliced
- ¼ tsp. of ground black pepper
- 2 tbsp. of soy sauce
- 2 tbsp. of oyster sauce
- 1 garlic clove, minced
- 2 tsp. of peeled and minced fresh ginger-root
- 2 spring onions, trimmed and sliced with white and green parts separated
- 110 g fresh mushrooms, divided
- 1 medium red bell pepper, membranes, and seeds removed
- 2 medium zucchinis (400g), cut, sliced

INSTRUCTIONS

1. In a skillet, heat one teaspoon vegetable oil over medium-high heat. Put the sliced chicken, season with black pepper, and cook until the chicken is completed (internal temperature about 165°F).

2. While the chicken cooks, prepare the sauce by combining the oyster sauce, soy sauce, and a couple of tablespoons of vegetable oil in a bowl and whisking together. Set aside.

3. With the same skillet used to cook the chicken, heat one teaspoon vegetable oil and put the garlic, ginger, and white onion pieces; cook until fragrant, about 1 minute. Put the mushrooms and bell peppers and still cook until just tender, about 3 minutes. Add zucchini noodles and toss to mix.

4. Pour in the sauce and put the chicken; cook until zucchini is tender and the mixture is heated for five minutes.

5. Garnish with green parts of spring onions.

Porridge with Walnuts

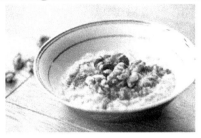

Prep Time: 10 mins **Cook Time:** 15 mins **Total Time:** 25 mins

MAKES 1 SERVINGS

INGREDIENTS

- ➢ 50 g raspberries
- ➢ 50 g blueberries
- ➢ 25 g of ground walnuts
- ➢ 20 g of crushed flaxseed
- ➢ 10 g of oatmeal
- ➢ 200 ml nut drink
- ➢ Agave syrup
- ➢ ½ teaspoon of cinnamon salt

INSTRUCTIONS

1. Warm the nut drink in a little saucepan.
2. Add the walnuts, flaxseed, and oatmeal, stirring constantly.
3. Stir in the cinnamon and salt.

4. Simmer for 8 minutes.

5. Keep stirring everything.

6. Sweet the entire thing.

7. Put the porridge in a bowl.

8. Wash the berries and allow them to drain.

9. Add them to the porridge and serve everything.

Walnut Crunch Banana Bread

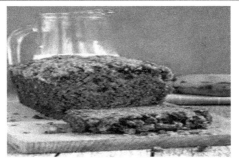

Prep Time: 5 mins **Cook Time:** 1 hr 30 mins   **Total Time:** 1 hr 30 mins

MAKES 1 SERVINGS

INGREDIENTS

- ➢ 4 ripe bananas
- ➢ 1/4 cup of maple syrup
- ➢ 1 tablespoon of apple cider vinegar
- ➢ 1 teaspoon of vanilla extract
- ➢ 11/2 cups of whole-wheat flour
- ➢ 1/2 teaspoon of ground cinnamon
- ➢ 1/2 teaspoon of baking soda
- ➢ 1/4 cup of walnut pieces (optional)

INSTRUCTIONS

1. Preheat the oven to 350°F.
2. In a large bowl, use a fork or mixing spoon to mash the bananas until they reach a puréed consistency. Stir in the

maple syrup, apple vinegar, and vanilla.

3. add the flour, cinnamon, and baking soda.

4. Gently pour the batter into a loaf pan, filling it no quite three-quarters of the way full. Bake it for 1 hour or until you can stick a knife into the center and it comes out clean.

5. Remove from the oven and allow cooling on the countertop for at least 30 minutes before serving.

Lean and Green Cicken Pesto Pasta

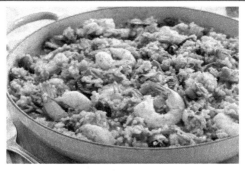

Prep Time: 5 mins **Cook Time:** 15 mins **Total Time:** 20 mins

MAKES 1 SERVINGS

INGREDIENTS

- ➤ 3 cups of raw kale leaves
- ➤ 2 tbsp. of olive oil
- ➤ 2 cups of fresh basil
- ➤ 1/4 teaspoon of salt
- ➤ 3 tbsp. of lemon juice
- ➤ Three garlic cloves
- ➤ 2 cups of cooked chicken breast
- ➤ 1 cup of baby spinach
- ➤ 6 ounce of uncooked chicken pasta
- ➤ 3 ounces of diced fresh mozzarella, basil leaves, or red pepper flakes to garnish

INSTRUCTIONS

1. Start by making the pesto, add the kale, lemon juice, basil, garlic cloves, olive oil, and salt to a blender and blend until it's smooth.

2. Add salt and pepper to taste. Cook the pasta and strain off the water. Reserve 1/4 cup of the liquid.

3. Get a bowl and blend everything, the cooked pasta, pesto, diced chicken, spinach, mozzarella, and the reserved pasta liquid.

4. Sprinkle the mixture with additional chopped basil or red paper flakes (optional).

5. Now your salad is prepared. You can serve it warm or chilled. Also, it is often taken as a salad mix-ins or as an entremot. Leftovers should be stored in the refrigerator inside an air-tight container for 3-5 days.

Zucchini Shrimp Scampi

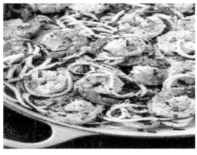

Prep Time: 15 mins **Cook Time:** 10 mins **Total Time:** 25 mins

MAKES 4 SERVINGS

INGREDIENTS

- ➢ 2 tablespoons unsalted butter
- ➢ 1 pound medium shrimp, peeled and deveined 3 cloves garlic, minced
- ➢ 1/2 teaspoon red pepper flakes, or more, to taste
- ➢ 1/4 cup chicken stock
- ➢ Juice of 1 lemon
- ➢ Kosher salt and freshly ground black pepper, to taste
- ➢ 1/2 pounds (4 medium-sized) zucchini, spiralized
- ➢ 2 tablespoons freshly grated Parmesan
- ➢ 2 tablespoons chopped fresh parsley leaves

INSTRUCTIONS

1. Melt butter in a large skillet over medium-high heat. Add shrimp, garlic, and red pepper flakes. Cook, stirring

occasionally, until pink, about 2-3 minutes.

2. Stir in chicken stock and lemon juice; season with salt and pepper, to taste. Bring to a simmer; stir in zucchini noodles until well combined, about 1-2 minutes.

3. Serve immediately, garnished with Parmesan and parsley, if desired.

Light Paprika Moussaka

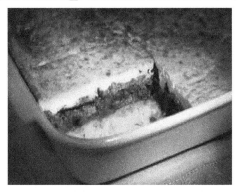

Prep Time: 15 mins **Cook Time:** 45 mins **Total Time:** 1hr

MAKES 3 SERVINGS

INGREDIENTS

- ➤ 1 eggplant, trimmed
- ➤ 1 cup of ground chicken
- ➤ 1/3 cup of white onion, diced
- ➤ 3 oz. Cheddar cheese, shredded
- ➤ 1 potato, sliced
- ➤ 1 teaspoon of olive oil
- ➤ 1 teaspoon of salt
- ➤ ½ cup of milk
- ➤ 1 tablespoon of butter
- ➤ 1 tablespoon of ground paprika
- ➤ 1 tablespoon of Italian seasoning
- ➤ 1 teaspoon of tomato paste

INSTRUCTIONS

1. Cut the eggplant lengthwise and dash with salt.
2. Dispense vegetable oil in the skillet and add sliced potato.
3. Roast potato for two minutes from all sides.
4. Then transfer it to the plate.
5. Put eggplant in the skillet and roast it for two minutes from all sides too.
6. Dispense milk in the pan and bring it to boil.
7. Add tomato paste, Italian seasoning, paprika, butter, and cheddar.
8. Then mix together onion with ground chicken.
9. Arrange the sliced potato in the casserole in one layer.
10. Then add ½ a part of all sliced eggplants.
11. Spread the eggplants with ½ part of the chicken mixture.
12. Then add remaining eggplants.
13. Pour the milk mixture over the eggplants.
14. Bake moussaka for 30 minutes at 355F.

Smoky Ribs in a BBQ Peach Sauce

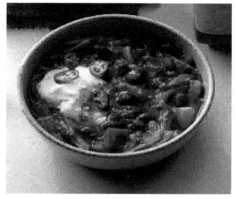

Prep Time: 5 mins **Cook Time:** 8 hr **Total Time:** 8 hr-5 mins

MAKES 4 SERVINGS

INGREDIENTS

- ➢ 1 red onion, chopped
- ➢ 2 pounds' of pork, ground
- ➢ 4 garlic cloves, minced
- ➢ 2 red bell peppers, chopped
- ➢ 1 celery stalk, chopped
- ➢ 25 ounces of fresh tomatoes, peeled, crushed
- ➢ ¼ cup of green chilies, chopped
- ➢ 2 tablespoons of fresh oregano, chopped
- ➢ 2 tablespoons of chili powder
- ➢ A pinch of salt and black pepper
- ➢ A drizzle of olive oil

INSTRUCTIONS

1. Heat up a sauté pan with the oil over medium-high heat and add the onion, garlic, and meat. Mix and brown for five minutes, then transfer to your slow cooker.
2. Add the rest of the ingredients, toss, cover, and cook on low for 8 hours.
3. Divide everything into bowls and serve.

Lemon Dill Trout

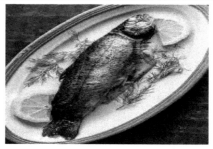

Prep Time: 5 mins **Cook Time:** 20 mins **Total Time:** 25 mins

MAKES 4 SERVINGS

INGREDIENTS

- ➤ 2 lb. of pan-dressed trout (or other small fish), fresh or frozen ½ tsp. salt
- ➤ ½ cup of butter or margarine
- ➤ 2 tbsp. of dill weed
- ➤ 3 tbsp. of lemon juice

INSTRUCTIONS

1. Cut the fish lengthwise and season it with pepper.
2. Prepare a skillet by melting the butter and dill.
3. Fry the fish on high heat, flesh side down, for 2-3 minutes per side.
4. Remove the fish. Add the juice to the butter and dill to make a sauce.
5. Serve the fish with the sauce.

Pancakes With Berries

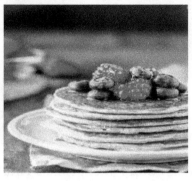

Prep Time: 5 mins **Cook Time:** 20 mins **Total Time:** 25 mins

MAKES 2 SERVINGS

INGREDIENTS

- 1 egg
- 50 g spelled flour
- 50 g almond flour
- 15 g coconut flour
- 150 ml of water
- salt

Filling:

- 40 g mixed berries
- 10 g chocolate
- 5 g powdered sugar
- 4 tbsp. of yogurt

INSTRUCTIONS

1. Put the flour, egg, and a pinch of salt in a blender jar.
2. Add 150 ml of water.
3. Mix everything with a whisk.
4. Mix everything into a batter.
5. Heat a coated pan.
6. Put in half the batter.
7. Once the pancake is firm, turn it over.
8. remove the pancake, add the last half of the batter to the pan and repeat.
9. Melt chocolate over a water bath.
10. Let the pancakes cool.
11. Brush the pancakes with the yogurt.
12. Wash the berry and let it drain.
13. Put berries on the yogurt.
14. Roll up the pancakes.
15. Sprinkle them with the granulated sugar.
16. Decorate the entire thing with the melted chocolate.

Yogurt with Granola and Persimmon

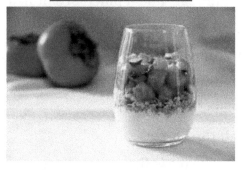

Prep Time: 5 mins **Cook Time:** 5 mins **Total Time:** 10 mins

MAKES 1 SERVINGS

INGREDIENTS

- ➤ 150g Greek-style yogurt
- ➤ 20g oatmeal
- ➤ 60g fresh persimmons
- ➤ 30 ml of tap water

INSTRUCTIONS

1. Put the oatmeal in the pan with no fat.
2. Toast them, constantly stirring, until golden brown.
3. Then, put them on a plate and allow them to calm down briefly.
4. Peel the persimmon and put it in a bowl with the water. Mix the entire thing into a fine puree.

5. Put the yogurt, the toasted oatmeal, and the puree in layers in a glass and serve.

Shake Cake Fueling

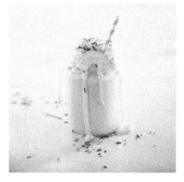

Prep Time: 5 mins **Cook Time:** 0 mins **Total Time:** 5 mins

MAKES 1 SERVINGS

INGREDIENTS

- ➤ 1/4 teaspoon of baking powder
- ➤ Two tablespoons of eggbeaters or egg whites
- ➤ Two tablespoons of water
- ➤ Other options that are not compulsory include sweeteners, reduced- fat cream cheese, etc.

INSTRUCTIONS

1. Begin by preheating the oven.
2. Mix all the ingredients; begin with the dry ingredients first before adding the wet ingredients.
3. After the mixture/batter is prepared, pour gently into muffin cups.
4. Inside the oven, place, and bake for about 16-18minutes

or until it's baked and prepared. Allow it to chill completely.

5. Add additional toppings of your choice and ensure your delicious shake cake is refreshing.

Mini Mac in a Bowl

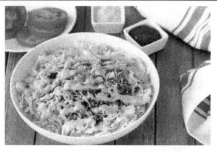

Prep Time: 5 mins **Cook Time:** 15 mins **Total Time:** 20 mins

MAKES 1 SERVINGS

INGREDIENTS

- ➤ 5 ounce of lean ground beef
- ➤ 2 tablespoons of diced white or yellow onion
- ➤ 1/8 teaspoon of onion powder
- ➤ 1/8 teaspoon of white vinegar
- ➤ 1 ounce of dill pickle slices
- ➤ One teaspoon sesame seed
- ➤ 3 cups of shredded Romaine lettuce
- ➤ Cooking spray
- ➤ 2 tablespoons reduced-fat shredded cheddar cheese
- ➤ 2 tablespoons of Wish-bone light thousand island as dressing

INSTRUCTIONS

1. Place a lightly greased small skillet ablaze to heat, Add

your onion to cook for about 2-3 minutes,

2. Next, add the meat and allow to cook until it's brown

3. Finally, top the lettuce with the cooked meat and sprinkle cheese on it; add your pickle slices.

4. Drizzle the mixture with the sauce and sprinkle the sesame seeds also. Your mini mac in a bowl is prepared for consumption.

Crunchy Quinoa Meal

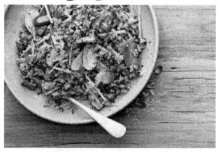

Prep Time: 5 mins **Cook Time:** 25 mins **Total Time:** 30 mins

MAKES 2 SERVINGS

INGREDIENTS

- ➢ 3 cups of coconut milk
- ➢ 1 cup of rinsed quinoa
- ➢ 1/8 tsp. of ground cinnamon
- ➢ 1 cup of raspberry
- ➢ 1/2 cup of chopped coconuts

INSTRUCTIONS

1. In a saucepan, pour milk and bring to an overboil at moderate heat. Add the quinoa to the milk, then bring it to a boil another time.
2. You then let it simmer for at least 15 minutes on medium heat until the milk is reduced.
3. Stir in the cinnamon, then mix properly.
4. Cover it, then cook for 8 minutes until the milk is totally

absorbed. Add the raspberry and cook the meal for 30 seconds.

5. Serve and enjoy.

Easy Chicken Soup

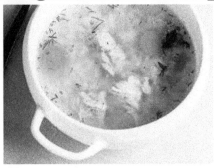

Prep Time: 10 mins **Cook Time:** 1 hr **Total Time:** 1 hr 10 mins

MAKES 4 SERVINGS

INGREDIENTS

- ➢ 2 cups of Shredded chicken, cooked
- ➢ 1 cup of Carrots, diced
- ➢ 1 cup Celery, diced
- ➢ 1 cup of Onion, diced
- ➢ 10 cups of Chicken broth
- ➢ 1 tablespoon of Italian seasoning
- ➢ 1 Bay leaf
- ➢ A dash of Sea salt
- ➢ A dash of Black pepper
- ➢ 1 Spaghetti squash

INSTRUCTIONS

1. Combine all the Ingredients: minus the spaghetti squash

in a pot over medium heat. Cook until it boils, then decrease to a simmer and cover the pot. Cook for one hour.

2. Next, preheat the oven to about 375 degrees F, then punch holes in the spaghetti squash with a knife. Send to a baking sheet and heat in the oven for sixty minutes.

3. When the spaghetti squash is cooked, cut in half and scoop out the strands using a fork. Remove the herb and add in half the spaghetti squash strands.

Low Carb Black Beans Chili Chicken

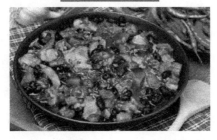

Prep Time: 10 mins **Cook Time:** 25 mins **Total Time:** 35 mins

MAKES 10 SERVINGS

INGREDIENTS

- 1-3/4 pounds of chicken breasts, cubed (boneless skinless)
- 2 sweet red peppers, chopped
- 1 onion, chopped
- 3 tablespoons of olive oil
- 1 can of chopped green chiles
- 4 cloves of garlic, minced
- 2 tablespoons of chili powder
- 2 teaspoons of ground cumin
- 1 teaspoon of ground coriander
- 2 cans of black beans, rinsed and drained
- 1 can of Italian stewed tomatoes, cut up
- 1 cup of chicken broth or beer
- 1/2 to 1 cup of water

INSTRUCTIONS

1. Put oil into a skillet and place over medium heat. Add in the red pepper, chicken, and onion and cook until the chicken is brown about five minutes.
2. Add in the garlic, chiles, chili powder, coriander, and cumin, and cook for an additional minute.
3. Next, add in the tomatoes, beans, half a cup of water, and broth and cook until it boils. Decrease the heat, uncover the skillet and cook while stirring for fifteen minutes.
4. Serve.

Yummy Smoked Salmon

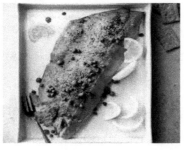

Prep Time: 10 mins **Cook Time:** 10 mins **Total Time:** 20 mins

MAKES 3 SERVINGS

INGREDIENTS

- ➢ 4 eggs; whisked
- ➢ 1/2 teaspoon of avocado oil
- ➢ 4 ounces of smoked salmon; chopped.

For the sauce:

- ➢ 1/2 cup of cashews; soaked; drained
- ➢ 1/4 cup of green onions; chopped.
- ➢ 1 teaspoon of garlic powder
- ➢ 1 cup of coconut milk
- ➢ 1 tablespoon of lemon juice
- ➢ Salt and black pepper to the taste

INSTRUCTIONS

1. In your blender machine, combine cashews with coconut

milk, garlic powder, and juice and blend well.

2. Put salt, pepper, and green onions, blend again well, send to a bowl, and confine the fridge for now.
3. Heat up a skillet with the oil over slight-low heat; put eggs, stir a little and cook until they are almost done
4. Put in your preheated broiler and cook until eggs set.
5. Divide eggs on plates, top with salmon, and serve with the scallion sauce on top.

Delicious Instant Pot Buffalo Chicken Soup

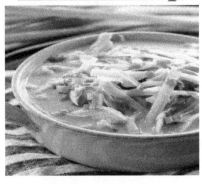

Prep Time: 10 mins **Cook Time:** 20 mins **Total Time:** 30 mins

MAKES 6 SERVINGS

INGREDIENTS

- 1 tablespoon of Olive oil
- 1/2 Onion, diced
- 1/2 cup of Celery, diced
- 4 cloves of Garlic, minced
- 1 lb. of Shredded chicken, cooked
- 4 cup of Chicken bone broth, or any chicken broth
- 3 tablespoons of Buffalo sauce
- 6 oz. of Cream cheese
- 1/2 cup of half & half

INSTRUCTIONS

1. Switch the instant pot to the sauté function. Add in the

chopped onion, oil, and celery. Cook till the onions are brown and translucent, about ten minutes.

2. Add in the garlic and cook until fragrant, about one minute. Switch off the instant pot.

3. Add in the broth, shredded chicken, and buffalo sauce. Cover the instant pot and seal. Switch the soup feature on and set the time to 5 minutes.

4. When cooked, release pressure naturally for five minutes, then quickly.

5. Scoop out one cup of the soup liquid into a blender bowl, then add in the cheese and blend until smooth. Pour the puree into the instant pot, then add in the half and half and stir to mix.

Yummy Mushroom Asparagus Frittata

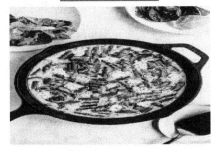

Prep Time: 25 mins **Cook Time:** 20 mins **Total Time:** 45 mins

MAKES 8 SERVINGS

INGREDIENTS

- 8 eggs
- 1/2 cup of whole-milk ricotta cheese
- 2 tablespoons of lemon juice
- 1/2 teaspoon of salt
- 1/4 teaspoon of pepper
- 1 tablespoon of olive oil
- 1 package of frozen asparagus spears, thawed
- 1 onion, halved and thinly sliced
- 1/4 cup of baby Portobello mushrooms, sliced
- 1/2 cup of sweet green or red pepper, finely choppe

INSTRUCTIONS

1. First, preheat the oven to about 300 and fifty degrees F,

then whisk the ricotta cheese, eggs, salt, lemon juice, and pepper in a bowl.

2. Pour oil into a skillet and add onion, asparagus, mushrooms, and red pepper. Cook until pepper and onions are tender, about eight minutes. Add in the egg mixture and transfer to the oven. Bake until eggs are set, about twenty-five minutes.

3. Keep aside to chill, then dig wedges.

Easiest Tuna Cobbler Ever

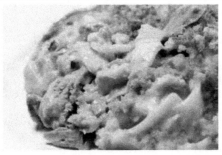

Prep Time: 15 mins **Cook Time:** 25 mins **Total Time:** 40 mins

MAKES 4 SERVINGS

INGREDIENTS

- ➤ Water, cold (1/3 cup)
- ➤ Tuna, canned, drained (10 ounces)
- ➤ Sweet pickle relish (2 tablespoons)
- ➤ Mixed vegetables, frozen (1 ½ cups)
- ➤ Soup, cream of chicken, condensed (10 ¾ ounces)
- ➤ Pimientos, sliced, drained (2 ounces)
- ➤ Lemon juice (1 teaspoon) Paprika

INSTRUCTIONS

1. Preheat the air fryer at 375 degrees Fahrenheit.
2. Mist cooking spray into a round casserole (1 ½ quart).
3. Mix the frozen vegetables with milk, soup, lemon juice, relish, pimientos, and tuna in a saucepan. Cook for 8 minutes over medium heat.

4. Fill the casserole with the tuna mixture.

5. Mix the biscuit mix with cold water to make a soft dough. Beat for half a moment before dropping by four spoonfuls into the casserole.

6. Dust the dish with paprika before air frying for 20 to 25 minutes.

Tuna Melts

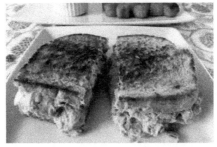

Prep Time: 15 mins **Cook Time:** 30 mins **Total Time:** 45 mins

MAKES 8 SERVINGS

INGREDIENTS

- ➤ Salt (1/8 teaspoon)
- ➤ Onion, chopped (1/3 cup)
- ➤ Biscuits, refrigerated, flaky layers (16 1/3 ounces)
- ➤ Tuna, water-packed, drained (10 ounces)
- ➤ Mayonnaise (1/3 cup) Pepper (1/8 teaspoon)
- ➤ Cheddar cheese, shredded (4 ounces)
- ➤ Tomato, chopped
- ➤ Sour cream
- ➤ Lettuce

INSTRUCTIONS

1. Preheat the air fryer at 325 degrees Fahrenheit.
2. Mist cooking spray onto a cooking sheet.
3. Mix tuna with mayonnaise, pepper, salt, and onion.

4. Separate dough so you have 8 biscuits; press each into 5-inch rounds.

5. Arrange 4 biscuit rounds on the sheet. Fill at the middle with tuna mixture before topping with cheese. Cover with the remaining biscuit rounds and press to seal.

6. Air-fry for fifteen to twenty minutes. Slice each sandwich into halves. Serve each bit topped with lettuce, tomato, and soured cream.

Potato Bacon Mush

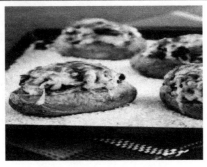

Prep Time: 10 mins **Cook Time:** 20 mins **Total Time:** 30 mins

MAKES 4 SERVINGS

INGREDIENTS

- ➢ 3 sweet potatoes, peeled
- ➢ 4 oz. of bacon, chopped
- ➢ 1 cup of chicken stock
- ➢ 1 tablespoon of butter
- ➢ teaspoon of salt
- ➢ oz. of Parmesan, grated

INSTRUCTIONS

1. Slice sweet potato and put it in the pot.
2. Add chicken stock and shut the lid.
3. Cook the vegetables for fifteen minutes or until they are soft. After this, drain the chicken stock.
4. Mash the sweet potato with the assistance of the potato masher. Add cheese and butter.

5. Mix salt and chopped bacon. Fry the mixture until it's crunchy (10-15 minutes).

6. Add cooked bacon in the mashed sweet potato and blend up with the assistance of the spoon.

7. It is recommended to serve the meal warm or hot.

Creamy Penne

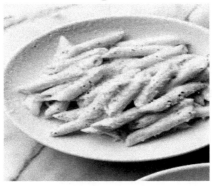

Prep Time: 10 mins **Cook Time:** 25 mins **Total Time:** 35 mins

MAKES 4 SERVINGS

INGREDIENTS

- ½ cup of penne, dried
- 9 oz. of chicken fillet
- 1 teaspoon of Italian seasoning
- 1 tablespoon of olive oil
- 1 tomato, chopped
- 1 cup of heavy cream
- 1 tablespoon of fresh basil, chopped
- ½ teaspoon of salt
- 2 oz. of Parmesan, grated
- 1 cup of water for cooking

INSTRUCTIONS

1. Pour water into the pan, add penne, and boil it for 15

minutes. Then drain water.

2. Dispense olive oil in the pan and heat it up.

3. Slice the chicken fillet and put it in the hot oil.

4. Sprinkle chicken with Italian seasoning and roast for two minutes from all sides.

5. Then add fresh basil, salt, tomato, and cheese.

6. Stir well.

7. Add cream and cooked penne.

8. Cook the meal for five minutes more over medium heat. Stir it from time to time.

Prosciutto Spinach Salad

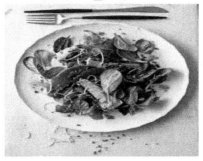

Prep Time: 5 mins **Cook Time:** 5 mins **Total Time:** 10 mins

MAKES 2 SERVINGS

INGREDIENTS

- ➤ 2 cups of baby spinach
- ➤ 1/3 lb. of prosciutto
- ➤ 1 cantaloupe
- ➤ 1 avocado
- ➤ ¼ cup of diced red onion handful of raw, unsalted walnuts

INSTRUCTIONS

1. Pour a cupful of spinach on each plate.
2. Top with the diced prosciutto, cubes of melon balls, slices of avocado, a couple of purple onions, and a couple of walnuts.
3. Add some freshly ground pepper, if you wish.
4. Serve!

Lattuce Salad with Beef Strips

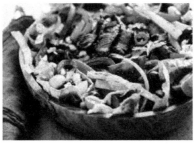

Prep Time: 10 mins **Cook Time**: 10 mins **Total Time:** 20 mins

MAKES 5 SERVINGS

INGREDIENTS

- 2 cup of lettuce
- 10 oz. of beef brisket
- 2 tablespoon of sesame oil
- 1 tablespoon of sunflower seeds
- 1 cucumber
- 1 teaspoon of ground black pepper
- 1 teaspoon of paprika
- 1 teaspoon of Italian spices
- 2 teaspoon of butter
- 1 teaspoon of dried dill
- 2 tablespoon of coconut milk

INSTRUCTIONS

1. Cut the meat brisket into strips. Sprinkle the meat strips

with the ground black pepper, paprika, and dried dill. Preheat the air fryer Put the butter in the air fryer basket tray and melt it. Then add the meat strips and cook them for six minutes on all sides.

2. Meanwhile, tear the lettuce and toss it in a big salad bowl. Crush the sunflower seeds and sprinkle them over the lettuce. Chop the cucumber into tiny cubes and increase the salad bowl.

3. Then combine the olive oil and Italian spices together. Stir the oil. Combine the lettuce mixture with the coconut milk and stir it using two wooden spatulas. When the meat is cooked – let it chill to room temperature.

4. Add the meat strips to the salad bowl. Stir it gently and sprinkle the salad with the vegetable oil dressing.

5. Serve the dish immediately.

Bell-Pepper Corn Wrapped in Tortilla

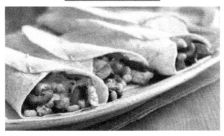

Prep Time: 5 mins **Cook Time:** 15 mins **Total Time:** 20 mins

MAKES 1 SERVINGS

INGREDIENTS

- ➢ 1/4 small red bell pepper, chopped
- ➢ 1/4 small yellow onion, diced
- ➢ 1/4 tablespoon of water
- ➢ 1/2 cobs grilled corn kernels
- ➢ One large tortilla
- ➢ One-piece commercial vegan nuggets, chopped
- ➢ Mixed greens for garnish

INSTRUCTIONS

1. Preparing the ingredients. Preheat the instant Crisp Air Fryer to 400°F.
2. In a skillet heated over medium heat, water sautés the vegan nuggets and the onions, bell peppers, and corn

kernels. Set aside. Place filling inside the corn tortillas. Air Frying.

3. Lock the air fryer lid. Fold the tortillas and place inside the instant Crisp Air Fryer and cook for 15 minutes until the tortilla wraps are crispy.

4. Serve with mixed greens on top.

Cheesy Cauliflower Fritters

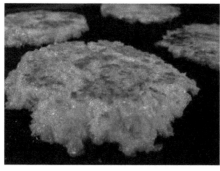

Prep Time: 10 mins **Cook Time:** 5 mins **Total Time:** 15 mins

MAKES 1 SERVINGS

INGREDIENTS

- ➢ 1/2 cup of chopped parsley
- ➢ 1 cup of Italian breadcrumbs
- ➢ 1/3 cup of shredded mozzarella cheese
- ➢ 1/3 cup of shredded sharp cheddar cheese
- ➢ One egg
- ➢ Two minced garlic cloves
- ➢ Three chopped scallions
- ➢ One head of cauliflower

INSTRUCTIONS

1. Preparing the Ingredients. Cut the cauliflower up into florets. Wash well and pat dry.
2. Place into a food processor and pulse 20-30 seconds till

it is like rice. Place the cauliflower rice in a bowl and blend with pepper, salt, egg, cheeses, breadcrumbs, garlic, and scallions.

3. With hands, form 15 patties of the mixture, then add more breadcrumbs if needed. Air Frying.

4. With olive oil, spritz patties, and put the fitters into your Instant Crisp Air Fryer. Pile it in a single layer.

5. Lock the air fryer lid. Set temperature to 390°F, and set time to 7 minutes, flipping after 7 minutes.

Coconut Battered Cauliflower Bites

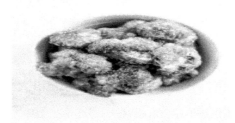

Prep Time: 5 mins **Cook Time:** 5 mins **Total Time:** 10 mins

MAKES 1 SERVINGS

INGREDIENTS

- ➤ Salt and pepper to taste
- ➤ One flax egg or one tablespoon flaxseed meal + 3 tablespoon water
- ➤ One small cauliflower, cut into florets
- ➤ One teaspoon of mixed spice
- ➤ 1/2 teaspoon of mustard powder
- ➤ Two tablespoons of maple syrup
- ➤ One clove of garlic, minced
- ➤ Two tablespoons of soy sauce
- ➤ 1/3 cup of oats flour
- ➤ 1/3 cup of plain flour
- ➤ 1/3 cup of desiccated coconut

INSTRUCTIONS

1. In a bowl, mix oats, flour, and desiccated coconut. Season with salt and pepper to taste. Set aside.

2. In another bowl, place the flax egg and add a pinch of salt to taste. Set aside. Season the cauliflower with mixed spice and mustard powder. Dredge the florets in the flax egg first, then in the flour mixture.

3. Air Frying. Place inside the instant Crisp Air Fryer, lock the air fryer lid, and cook at 400°F or 15 minutes.

4. Meanwhile, place the maple syrup, garlic, and soy sauce in a saucepan and heat over medium flame.

5. Turn it to a boil and adjust the heat to low until the sauce thickens.

6. After 15 minutes, remove the instant Crisp Air Fryer's florets and place them in the saucepan. T

7. Oss to coat the florets and place inside the instant Crisp Air Fryer, and cook for an additional 5 minutes.

Sunflower Parmesan Cheese

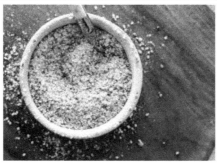

Prep Time: 5 mins **Cook Time:** 30 mins **Total Time:** 35 mins

MAKES 1 SERVINGS

INGREDIENTS

- ➤ 1/2 cup of sunflower seeds
- ➤ 2 tablespoons of nutritional yeast
- ➤ 1/2 teaspoon of garlic powder

INSTRUCTIONS

1. In a food processor or blender, combine the sunflower seeds, nutritional yeast, and garlic powder.
2. Process on low for 30 to 45 seconds, or until the sunflower seeds are weakened to the size of coarse sea salt.
3. Store in a safe refrigerator container for up to 2 months.

Crackpot Chicken Taco Soup

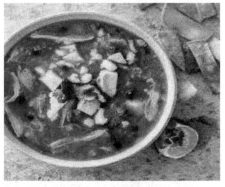

Prep Time: 15 mins **Cook Time:** 6 hr **Total Time:** 6 hr 15 mins

MAKES 6 SERVINGS

INGREDIENTS

- ➤ 2 frozen boneless chicken breast
- ➤ 2 cans of white beans or black beans
- ➤ 1 can of diced tomatoes
- ➤ Green chili's
- ➤ 1/2 onion chopped
- ➤ 1/2 packet of taco seasoning
- ➤ 1/2 teaspoon of Garlic salt
- ➤ 1 cup of chicken broth
- ➤ Salt and pepper to taste
- ➤ Tortilla chips, sour cheese cream, and cilantro as toppings, as well as chili pepper (this is optional).

INSTRUCTIONS

1. Put your frozen chicken into the Crock-Pot and place the opposite ingredients into the pool too.

2. Leave to cook for about 6-8 hours. After cooking, remove the chicken and shred it to the size you would like.

3. Finally, place the shredded chicken into the crockpot and put it on a slow cooker. Stir and allow to cook.

4. You can add more beans and tomatoes also to assist stretch the meat and make it tastier.

Cream of Thyme Soup

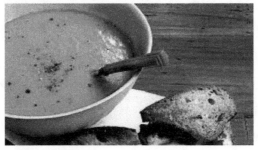

Prep Time: 5 mins **Cook Time:** 20 mins **Total Time:** 25 mins

MAKES 6 SERVINGS

INGREDIENTS

- 2 tbsp. of ghee
- 2 large red onions, diced
- 1/2 cup of raw cashew nuts, diced
- 2 (28 oz.) cans of tomatoes
- 1 tsp. of fresh thyme leaves + extra to garnish
- 1 1/2 cups of water
- Salt and black pepper to taste

INSTRUCTIONS

1. Melt ghee in a pot over medium heat and sauté the onions for 4 minutes until softened.
2. Stir in the tomatoes, thyme, water, cashews, and season with salt and black pepper.
3. Cover and bring to simmer for 10 minutes until

thoroughly cooked.

4. Open, turn the heat off, and puree the ingredients with an immersion blender. Adjust to taste and stir in the cream.

5. Spoon into soup bowls and serve.

Vegetables in Air Fryer

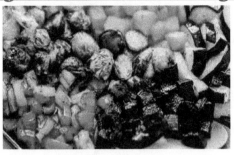

Prep Time: 20 mins **Cook Time:** 30 mins **Total Time:** 50 mins

MAKES 2 SERVINGS

INGREDIENTS

- ➢ 2 potatoes
- ➢ 1 zucchini
- ➢ 1 onion
- ➢ 1 red pepper
- ➢ 1 green pepper

INSTRUCTIONS

1. Cut the potatoes into slices. Cut the onion into rings.
2. Cut the zucchini slices.
3. Cut the peppers into strips.
4. Put all the ingredients in the bowl and add a little salt, ground pepper, and a few extra virgin vegetable oil drops.
5. Mix well. Pass to the basket of the air fryer. Select 1600C,

30 minutes.

6. Check that the vegetables are to your liking.

Fennel and Arugula Salad with Fig Vinaigrette

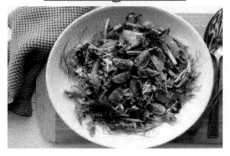

Prep Time: 15 mins **Cook Time:** 10 mins **Total Time:** 25 mins

MAKES 6 SERVINGS

INGREDIENTS

- ➢ 5 Ounces of washed and dried arugula
- ➢ 1 small fennel bulb, it can be either shaved or tiny sliced.
- ➢ 2 tablespoons of extra virgin oil or any cooking oil
- ➢ 1 teaspoon of lemon zest
- ➢ 1/2 teaspoon of salt _ Pepper (freshly ground)
- ➢ Pecorino

INSTRUCTIONS

1. Mix the arugula and shaved fennel in a serving bowl.
2. In another bowl, mix the olive oil or vegetable oil, lemon peel, salt, and pepper.
3. Shake together until it becomes creamy and smooth.

4. Pour and dress over the salad, tossing gently for it to mix.

5. Peel or shave out some slices of pecorino and put it on top of the salad

Mixed Potato Gratin

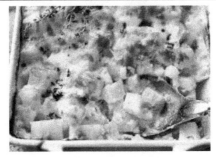

Prep Time: 20 mins **Cook Time:** 5 hr **Total Time:** 5 hr 20 mins

MAKES 4 SERVINGS

INGREDIENTS

- ➤ 6 Yukon Gold potatoes, thinly sliced
- ➤ 3 sweet potatoes, peeled and thinly sliced
- ➤ 2 onions, thinly sliced
- ➤ 4 garlic cloves, minced
- ➤ 3 tablespoons of whole-wheat flour
- ➤ 4 cups of 2% milk, divided
- ➤ 11/2 cups of Roasted Vegetable Broth
- ➤ 3 tablespoons of melted butter
- ➤ 1 teaspoon of dried thyme leaves
- ➤ 11/2 cups of shredded Havarti cheese

INSTRUCTIONS

1. Grease a 6-quart slow cooker with straight vegetable oil.
2. In the slow cooker, layer the potatoes, onions, and garlic.

3. In a large bowl, mix the flour with 1/2 cup of the milk until well combined.

4. Gradually add the remaining milk, stirring with a wire whisk to avoid lumps. Stir in the vegetable broth, melted butter, and thyme leaves.

5. Pour the milk mixture over the potatoes in the slow cooker and top with the cheese.

6. Cover and cook on low for 4 to 6 hours, or until the potatoes are tender when pierced with a fork.

Mexican Cauliflower Rice

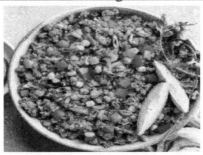

Prep Time: 10 mins **Cook Time:** 15 mins **Total Time:** 25 mins

MAKES 4 SERVINGS

INGREDIENTS

- head cauliflower, riced
- 1 tbsp olive oil
- 1 medium white onion, finely diced
- 2 cloves garlic, minced
- 1 jalapeno, seeded and minced
- 3 tbsp tomato paste
- 1 tsp sea salt
- 1 tsp cumin
- 1/2 tsp paprika
- 3 tbsp fresh chopped cilantro
- 1 tbsp lime juice

INSTRUCTIONS

1. Rice the cauliflower. Slice the florets from the head of the

cauliflower.

2. Fit a food processor with the s-blade.

3. Place half the florets into the bowl of the food processor and pulse until riced, scraping down the sides once halfway through to catch any larger pieces.

4. Scrape out the riced cauliflower and repeat with the remaining florets. Heat a skillet over medium-high heat. Add the oil and heat until it shimmers.

5. Add the onion and saute until soft and translucent, stirring occasionally, 5-6 minutes.

6. Add the garlic and jalapeno and saute until fragrant, 1-2 minutes.

7. Add the tomato paste, salt, cumin, and paprika and stir into the vegetables. Add the cauliflower rice and stir continuously until all ingredients are incorporated.

8. Continue sautéing, stirring occasionally, until the cauliflower releases its liquid and is dry and fluffy.

9. Remove the Mexican cauliflower rice from heat. Stir in the cilantro and lime juice.

10. Serve immediately.

Roasted Potatoes with Bacon

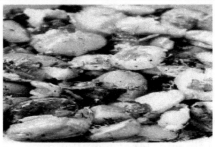

Prep Time: 10 mins **Cook Time:** 35 mins **Total Time:** 45 mins

MAKES 6 SERVINGS

INGREDIENTS

- ➢ 2 pounds red potatoes Yukon Gold or Russets work well too
- ➢ 1 pound Brussels sprouts
- ➢ 1/4 cup olive oil
- ➢ 3 cloves garlic minced
- ➢ 1 teaspoon rosemary optional
- ➢ 1 teaspoon kosher salt
- ➢ 1/2 teaspoon ground black pepper
- ➢ 1/2 pound bacon lightly cooked and cut into pieces

INSTRUCTIONS

1. Preheat oven to 400 degrees.
2. Scrub and rinse the potatoes. Pat dry and dice into one-inch pieces.

3. Wash Brussels sprouts and trim off the ends, slice in half length- wise. Whisk olive oil, garlic, rosemary (optional), salt, and pepper in a large bowl until well combined.

4. Add potatoes and Brussels sprouts and stir until potatoes and Brussels are coated in the oil mixture.

5. Place potatoes and Brussels sprouts on a baking sheet and sprinkle bacon pieces over the top.

6. Roast for 35-40 minutes.

7. Potatoes should be golden and soft and Brussels should be well roasted and lightly charred-- bacon should be nice and crispy.

Vegetarian Chili

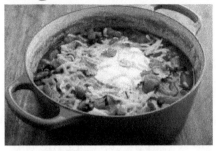

Prep Time: 10 mins **Cook Time:** 45 mins **Total Time:** 55 mins

MAKES 4 SERVINGS

INGREDIENTS

- ➤ 2 tablespoons olive oil
- ➤ 1 small yellow onion, diced (1 cup)
- ➤ 1 tablespoon minced garlic (reduce depending on garlic sensitivity)
- ➤ 1 red bell pepper, diced (heaping cup)
- ➤ 2 tablespoons ground chili powder
- ➤ 1/2 tablespoon dried (NOT ground) oregano
- ➤ 1 teaspoon ground cumin
- ➤ 1/2 teaspoon EACH: dried basil, seasoned salt, cayenne pepper, paprika 1/4 teaspoon cracked pepper
- ➤ 1/2 tablespoon white sugar
- ➤ 2 cans (14.5 ounces EACH) fire-roasted diced tomatoes
- ➤ 2 cans (14.5 ounces EACH) black beans, drained and rinsed

- 1 can (14.5 ounces) pinto beans, drained and rinsed
- 1 can (4 ounces) fire-roasted diced green chiles, optional
- 1 cup frozen corn
- 1 cup vegetable stock (vegetable broth will work)
- 1 bay leaf
- 2 tablespoons fresh lime juice
- Toppings: cheddar cheese, fat-free sour cream, avocado, cilantro, chives, tortilla strips, etc.

INSTRUCTIONS

1. Place a large heavy-bottomed pot (or dutch oven) over medium heat.
2. Pour in the olive oil and wait until shimmering, about 20 seconds.
3. Add in the diced onion and stir for 3-4 minutes. Add in the diced pepper and cook these veggies, stirring occasionally, until they are all very tender, about 6-9 minutes.
4. While the veggies are getting soft, mince the garlic and measure out all your spices, combining them into a small bowl: the chili powder, oregano, cumin, dried basil, salt, cayenne pepper, paprika, pepper, and sugar.
5. Stir together and set aside until onion/pepper are tender. Add in the garlic and all the seasonings you've already measured and set aside.

6. Cook, stirring constantly, until the seasonings and garlic are fragrant, about 45 seconds - 1 minute.

7. Be careful to not burn. Carefully add in the UNDRAINED diced tomatoes (they might sizzle splatter up a bit) and stir. Add in the drained and rinsed black beans, drained and rinsed pinto beans, chiles (if desired), frozen corn, and vegetable stock. Add in the bay leaf.

8. Stir to combine everything. Reduce the heat as needed to maintain a gentle simmer, and stir occasionally, for 25-30 minutes. Remove 1 and 1/2 cups of the chili and transfer to a blender. To avoid a mess, remove your blender lid's center insert and hold a kitchen towel firmly over the top.

9. Ensure the lid is securely fashioned and blend while holding the towel. Once smooth, pour this mixture back into your chili.

10. Stir to combine.

11. Add fresh lime and fresh cilantro as desired. Season to taste (I always add in a little bit more salt & pepper).

12. Garnish individual bowls with everyone's favorite toppings.

Balsamic Roast Beef

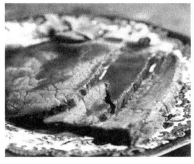

Prep Time: 5 mins **Cook Time:** 4 hr **Total Time**: 4 hr 5 mins

MAKES 4 SERVINGS

INGREDIENTS

- ➢ 1 (3-4 pound) boneless roast beef (chuck or round roast)
- ➢ 1 cup beef stock or broth
- ➢ 1/2 cup balsamic vinegar
- ➢ 1 tablespoon Worcestershire sauce
- ➢ 1 tablespoon soy sauce
- ➢ 1 tablespoon honey
- ➢ 1/2 teaspoon red pepper flakes
- ➢ 4 cloves garlic chopped

INSTRUCTIONS

1. Place roast beef into the insert of your slow cooker.
2. In a 2-cup measuring cup, mix all remaining ingredients.
3. Pour over roast beef and set the timer for your slow

cooker. (4 hours on High or 6-8 hours on Low).

4. Once roast beef has cooked, remove it from the slow cooker with tongs into a serving dish.

5. Break apart lightly with two forks and then ladle about 1/4 - 1/2 cup of gravy over roast beef.

6. Store remaining gravy in an airtight container in the refrigerator for another use.

Zucchini Boats

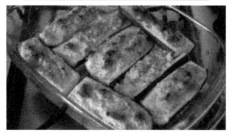

Prep Time: 10 mins **Cook Time:** 30 mins **Total Time:** 40 mins

MAKES 3 SERVINGS

INGREDIENTS

- ➢ 3 zucchinis
- ➢ 3/4 lb. chicken breast cut into cubes
- ➢ 1 Tbsp olive oil
- ➢ 1/4 tsp Italian seasoning
- ➢ 1/4 tsp garlic powder
- ➢ 1/4 tsp salt
- ➢ 1/4 tsp ground black pepper
- ➢ 3/4 cup pasta sauce
- ➢ 1/4 cup grated parmesan cheese
- ➢ 1/4 cup shredded mozzarella cheese

INSTRUCTIONS

1. Preheat oven to 400°F.
2. To prepare the zucchini, cut the zucchini in half lengthwise, then use a spoon or melon baller to scoop the

center flesh and seeds from the zucchini.

3. Repeat for the remaining zucchini.

4. Place the zucchini in a baking dish or cookie sheet cut-side up and lightly coat with cooking spray.

5. Place in the preheated oven for 15 minutes until the zucchini cooks slightly and becomes tender.

6. Meanwhile, to prepare the chicken, heat the olive oil in a large non-stick skillet over medium-high heat. Add the chicken along with the seasoning, salt, and pepper. Cook for 8-10 minutes until the chicken is cooked through.

7. Add the pasta sauce and cook for an additional 2 minutes, stirring occasionally. Scoop the chicken mixture into the zucchini boats.

8. Top the chicken with parmesan cheese and mozzarella cheese. Return the zucchini boats to the oven for 5 more minutes, or until the cheese is melted.

9. Sprinkle with fresh basil and parmesan cheese, if desired, and serve.

Creamed Spinach

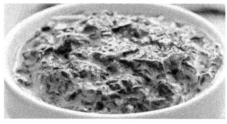

Prep Time: 5 mins **Cook Time:** 15 mins **Total Time:** 20 mins

MAKES 6 SERVINGS

INGREDIENTS

- ➢ 20-24 ounces fresh spinach (about 1 1/2 pounds)
- ➢ 5 tablespoons butter
- ➢ 1 onion finely chopped
- ➢ 4 cloves garlic crushed
- ➢ 1/4 cup flour
- ➢ 2 cups half and half (or whole milk)
- ➢ Kosher salt to taste
- ➢ black pepper to taste
- ➢ 1/2 cup Parmesan cheese (fresh, shredded-- not the powdered kind)
- ➢ 1/2 cup Mozzarella cheese
- ➢ 5 wedges Creamy Swiss

INSTRUCTIONS

1. Bring a large stockpot of water to a boil.

2. Add spinach and cook down for about 2-3 minutes or until spinach is wilted but not soggy.

3. Drain spinach well and then wring out using cheesecloth (preferred) or a kitchen towel. You can also press spinach in a fine- mesh strainer to try and remove excess water.

4. Set spinach aside.

5. In a large skillet over medium heat, melt butter.

6. Add onions and garlic and cook until onions become soft and transparent. Sprinkle flour over the onions and stir until flour is cooked (about 3 minutes).

7. Pour in half and half a little at a time, whisking constantly making a bechamel sauce. You want it to be the consistency of a thin gravy.

8. Add more half and a half or milk if needed. Add salt and pepper to taste. Add spinach and stir until spinach is well mixed in. Add Parmesan cheese, Mozzarella cheese, and creamy Swiss cheese (or cream cheese).

9. Stir until all cheeses are melted and completely mixed in.

10. Serve immediately.

Feta Salad

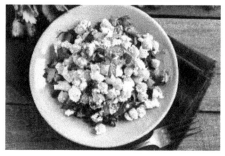

Prep Time: 15 mins **Cook Time:** 0 mins **Total Time:** 15 mins

MAKES 6 SERVINGS

INGREDIENTS

- ➢ 3 pounds watermelon cut into cubes
- ➢ 24 ounces blueberries
- ➢ 2 cucumbers sliced and quartered
- ➢ 8 ounces feta cheese cut into cubes
- ➢ 10 mint leaves sliced
- ➢ 5 basil leaves sliced
- ➢ 2 limes
- ➢ Salt to taste

INSTRUCTIONS

1. In a large bowl, combine watermelon, blueberries, cucumbers, and feta cheese.
2. Add mint, basil, and the juice from both limes. (Optional: add the zest from the limes as well).

3. Sprinkle with salt if desired.

4. Stir until all ingredients are coated in lime juice.

5. Chill until ready to serve.

Lemon Spaghetti

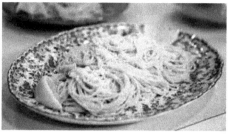

Prep Time: 5 mins **Cook Time:** 10 mins **Total Time:** 15 mins

MAKES 6 SERVINGS

INGREDIENTS

- ➤ 16 ounces spaghetti
- ➤ 2 lemons
- ➤ 1/2 cup olive oil
- ➤ 1/2 cup grated Parmesan cheese
- ➤ 3/4 teaspoon salt more to taste if needed
- ➤ Ground black pepper to taste
- ➤ 1/4 cup chopped
- ➤ fresh basil

INSTRUCTIONS

1. Cook spaghetti according to package directions. Reserve 1 cup of the pasta water and drain the rest from the spaghetti.
2. While pasta is cooking, zest, and juice the lemons. You

should get about 1/2 cup of lemon juice. If not, fill up the rest of the 1/2 cup with bottled lemon juice.

3. In a small bowl, add lemon juice, olive oil, parmesan, salt, and pepper. Whisk until combined.

4. Toss spaghetti with the lemon sauce until it is evenly coated. Add lemon zest and basil.

5. Add the reserved pasta water a little at a time until the sauce clings to the pasta and thickens a little.

6. Top with more fresh basil, lemon zest, parmesan, salt, and pepper. Serve hot.

Medterranean Pork Loin With Sun-Dried Tomatoes and Olives

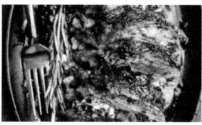

Prep Time: 10 mins **Cook Time:** 3 hr **Total Time:** 3 hr 10 mins

MAKES 4 SERVINGS

INGREDIENTS

- 11/2-2 lbs pork tenderloin
- 1 C Broth of your choice (chicken, vegetable, etc.)
- 2 teaspoons Garlic, chives, lemon, salt, pepper, onion, and garlic powder
- 1/2 teaspoon s Mediterranean Seasoning
- 10 green olives, sliced
- 1 T sun-dried tomatoes (not in oil) sliced thin

INSTRUCTIONS

1. Place pork loin in the bottom of the Crock-Pot (slow cooker.) Pour the broth over the meat.
2. Sprinkle with the seasonings, then scatter the olives and sun-dried tomatoes around the meat.
3. Place the lid on and cook on high for 4 hours, or low for

6 hours. Meat may need longer if frozen. It will be done when the internal temperature reaches 155 degrees F.

4. Slice the meat thin, drizzle with some of the broth, and garnish with a few olive and sun-dried tomato pieces.

5. Serve hot.

Bruschetta Chicken

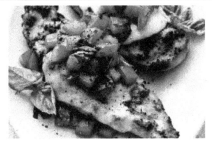

Prep Time: 10 mins **Cook Time:** 3 hr **Total Time:**3 hr 10 mins

MAKES 4 SERVINGS

INGREDIENTS

Chicken

- ➢ 2 tbsp olive oil, extra virgin
- ➢ 4 chicken breasts s
- ➢ alt & pepper to taste
- ➢ 1 tbsp dried basil
- ➢ 1 tbsp minced garlic

Bruschetta

- ➢ 3 ripe Roma tomatoes, diced
- ➢ 7 basil leaves, chopped
- ➢ 1 sprig oregano, chopped
- ➢ 2 tsp minced garlic
- ➢ 1 tbsp olive oil, extra virgin
- ➢ 1 tsp balsamic vinegar

- ➢ 1/4 tsp salt
- ➢ 1/4 tsp pepper

Balsamic Glaze

- ➢ 1 cup balsamic vinegar

INSTRUCTIONS

Chicken

1. Add olive oil to saute pan or cast-iron skillet. Heat pan to medium- high heat.
2. Add chicken to the hot pan. Sprinkle salt, pepper, and dried basil on top of each cutlet. Cook until browned, about 5 minutes. Flip chicken. Add garlic to the pan. Cook until the remaining side of the chicken is browned, about 5 minutes.

Bruschetta

1. Add all ingredients to a bowl and stir together until combined. Pour over your cooked chicken breasts.

Balsamic Glaze

1. Add 1 cup balsamic vinegar to a small saucepan.
2. Bring to a boil over medium-high heat.
3. Reduce heat to medium. You should see bubbling along

the outside of your pan.

4. Let simmer for 10 minutes. Stir occasionally as vinegar begins to thicken and coat the spoon.

5. Remove from heat and set aside to cool for a few minutes.

6. It will thicken a bit more as it sits and you'll end up with around 1/4 cup of balsamic glaze.

7. Drizzle over bruschetta topped chicken.

CPSIA information can be obtained
at www.ICGtesting.com
Printed in the USA
BVHW051554090321
602118BV00004B/364